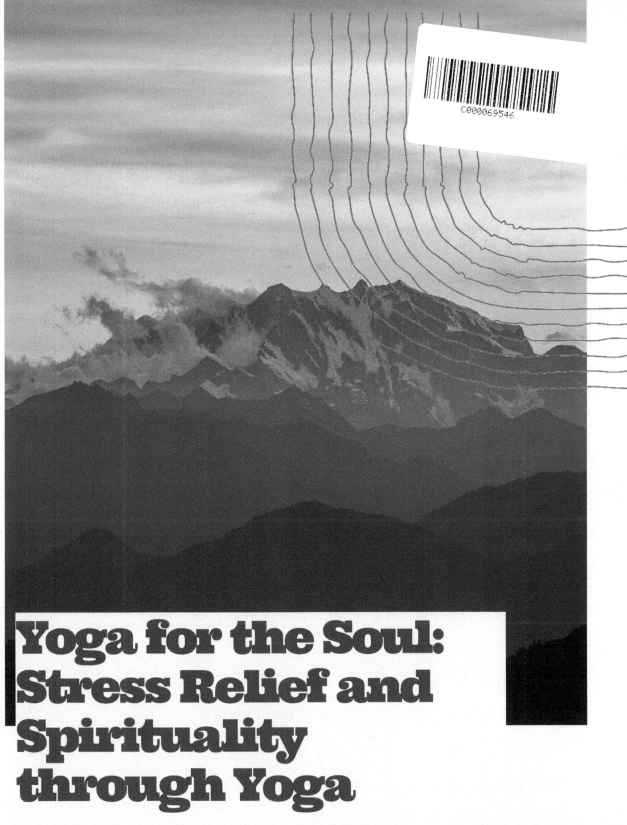

# Yoga for the Soul: Stress Relief and Spirituality through Yoga

How to Build Good Habits and Break Bad Ones

# Table Of Contents

Chapter 1: The Basics of Yoga                                          3

    The History of Yoga                                           4

    The Benefits of Yoga                                          4

    Different Types of Yoga Practices                             5

Chapter 2: Yoga for Stress Relief                                      8

    Understanding Stress and its Effects                          9

    Techniques for Managing Stress through Yoga                   9

    Incorporating Meditation and Mindfulness into Your

Practice                                                              11

Chapter 3: Yoga for Spirituality                                      13

    Connecting Mind, Body, and Spirit through Yoga               14

    Cultivating a Deeper Sense of Self-Awareness                 15

    Finding Inner Peace and Harmony through Yoga                 16

Chapter 4: Specialized Yoga Practices                                18

    Hot Yoga: Benefits and Precautions                           19

    Aerial Yoga: Taking Your Practice to New Heights             20

Restorative Yoga: Relaxing and Rejuvenating the Body                    21

Chapter 5: Yoga for Different Audiences                                 24

Yoga for Seniors: Gentle and Safe Practices                            25

Yoga for Children: Fun and Playful Poses                               26

Prenatal Yoga: Nurturing the Body and Baby                            27

Yoga for Beginners: Building a Strong Foundation                      27

Chapter 6: Advanced Yoga Practices                                     30

Vinyasa Yoga: Flowing Sequences for Strength and
Flexibility                                                            31

Yoga for Athletes: Enhancing Performance and
Preventing Injuries                                                    32

Chapter 7: Maintaining a Regular Yoga Practice                         34

Setting Realistic Goals and Intentions                                35

Overcoming Challenges and Plateaus                                    36

Creating a Sacred Space for Your Practice                             37

Chapter 8: The Spiritual Journey of Yoga                               39

Embracing the Present Moment with Mindfulness                         40

Cultivating a Sense of Gratitude and Compassion                      41

Finding Peace and Harmony Within Yourself and the
World                                                                  42

01

# Chapter 1: The Basics of Yoga

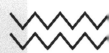

# The History of Yoga

Yoga has a rich and ancient history that dates back thousands of years. Its origins can be traced back to the Indus Valley civilization in India, where the practice was developed as a way to achieve spiritual enlightenment and oneness with the universe. The word "yoga" itself comes from the Sanskrit word "yuj," which means to yoke or unite, symbolizing the union of body, mind, and spirit.

Over the centuries, yoga has evolved and taken on many different forms and styles. From the traditional Hatha yoga to the more modern variations like Hot yoga, Aerial yoga, and Restorative yoga, there is a practice to suit every individual's needs and preferences. Each style of yoga has its own unique benefits and can be tailored to specific goals, whether it be stress relief, flexibility, strength, or mindfulness.

Yoga is not just a physical practice, but a spiritual one as well. It is a way to connect with our inner selves and find peace and tranquility amidst the chaos of daily life. Through meditation, breathwork, and mindful movement, yoga allows us to quiet the mind and tap into our true essence.

Today, yoga has become a popular practice worldwide, with millions of people reaping its numerous benefits. It is not just for the young and fit, but for people of all ages and abilities. From seniors looking to maintain flexibility and mobility, to children learning to focus and relax, to athletes seeking to improve their performance, there is a style of yoga for everyone.

Whether you are a beginner looking to start your yoga journey or a seasoned practitioner looking to deepen your practice, yoga has something to offer for everyone. It is a path to self-discovery, healing, and spiritual growth, and a powerful tool for stress relief and overall well-being. So why not roll out your mat and start your yoga journey today?

# The Benefits of Yoga

Yoga is not just a physical practice; it has numerous benefits for the mind, body, and soul. In this subchapter, we will explore the many advantages of incorporating yoga into your daily routine.

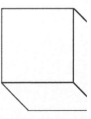

One of the most prominent benefits of yoga is stress relief. Through mindful breathing and gentle movements, yoga helps to calm the mind and reduce stress levels. This can be especially beneficial for those in today's fast-paced world who are constantly under pressure. Yoga is also a powerful tool for increasing spirituality and mindfulness. By connecting with your breath and body, you can tap into a sense of inner peace and tranquility. This can lead to a deeper understanding of yourself and the world around you.

For those who practice meditation or Zen, yoga can be a complementary practice that enhances your spiritual journey. The focus on being present in the moment and letting go of distractions can help you achieve a state of mindfulness that is essential for spiritual growth.

Additionally, yoga is a versatile practice that can be adapted to suit individuals of all ages and fitness levels. Whether you are a senior looking to improve flexibility, an athlete seeking to enhance performance, or a beginner just starting out on your yoga journey, there is a style of yoga that is perfect for you.

In conclusion, the benefits of yoga are vast and far-reaching. By incorporating yoga into your life, you can experience improved physical health, mental clarity, and spiritual growth. So why not roll out your mat and start reaping the rewards of this ancient practice today?

# Different Types of Yoga Practices

In the world of yoga, there are many different types of practices that cater to various needs and preferences. Whether you are looking to strengthen your body, calm your mind, or find spiritual enlightenment, there is a style of yoga that is perfect for you. In this subchapter, we will explore some of the most popular types of yoga practices and the benefits they offer.

Hot yoga, also known as Bikram yoga, is a practice that takes place in a heated room. The heat helps to loosen muscles and increase flexibility, making it a great option for those looking to improve their physical strength and endurance. Aerial yoga, on the other hand, involves practicing yoga poses while suspended from a hammock. This type of yoga can help improve balance, core strength, and overall flexibility.

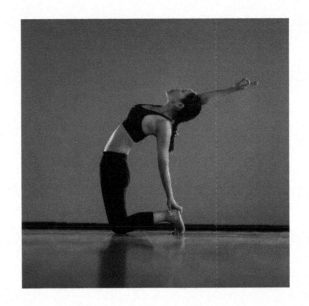

Restorative yoga is a gentle and relaxing practice that focuses on deep stretching and breathing exercises. It is perfect for those looking to reduce stress and improve their overall well-being. Yoga for seniors is tailored to the needs of older adults, with a focus on gentle movements and poses that help improve flexibility and balance.

Vinyasa yoga is a dynamic and flowing practice that links breath with movement. It is a great option for those looking to improve their cardiovascular fitness and build strength. Yoga for athletes focuses on improving performance and preventing injuries through a combination of strength, flexibility, and mindfulness practices. No matter your age, fitness level, or goals, there is a type of yoga practice that is perfect for you. By exploring different styles and finding what resonates with you, you can experience the many physical, mental, and spiritual benefits that yoga has to offer.

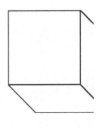

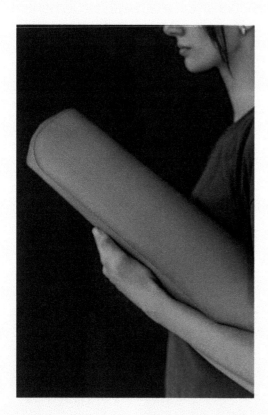

02

# Chapter 2: Yoga for Stress Relief

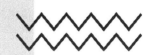

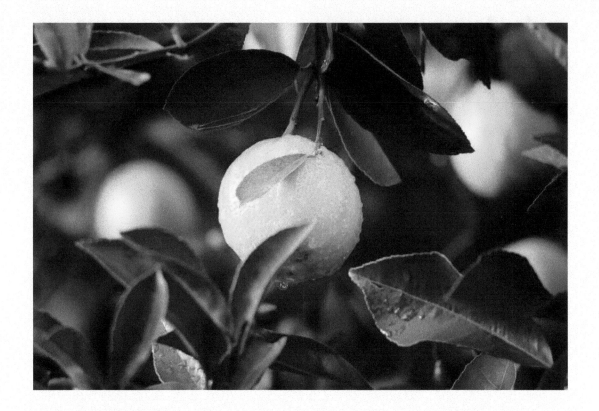

# Understanding Stress and its Effects

# Techniques for Managing Stress through Yoga

In today's fast-paced world, stress has become an inevitable part of our daily lives. However, managing stress is crucial for our overall well-being and spiritual growth. Yoga, with its focus on breath control, meditation, and physical postures, has been proven to be an effective tool for stress relief. In this subchapter, we will explore some techniques for managing stress through yoga.

One of the most powerful ways to manage stress through yoga is through deep breathing exercises. By focusing on the breath and practicing pranayama techniques, we can calm the mind and reduce stress levels. Incorporating deep, slow breathing into our yoga practice can help us stay present and centered, even in the midst of chaos.

Another effective technique for managing stress through yoga is through the practice of mindfulness. By being fully present in each moment and paying attention to our thoughts and emotions without judgment, we can cultivate a sense of inner peace and tranquility. Mindfulness can help us become more aware of our stress triggers and develop healthier coping mechanisms.

In addition to deep breathing and mindfulness, practicing physical postures (asanas) can also help us release tension and stress from the body. Restorative yoga, in particular, focuses on gentle, supported poses that promote relaxation and rejuvenation. By incorporating restorative poses into our yoga practice, we can activate the body's natural relaxation response and reduce stress hormones.

Overall, yoga offers a holistic approach to managing stress by addressing the mind, body, and spirit. By incorporating deep breathing, mindfulness, and physical postures into our yoga practice, we can cultivate a sense of inner peace and spiritual well-being. Whether you are a beginner or an experienced yogi, incorporating these techniques into your practice can help you find relief from stress and connect more deeply with your true self.

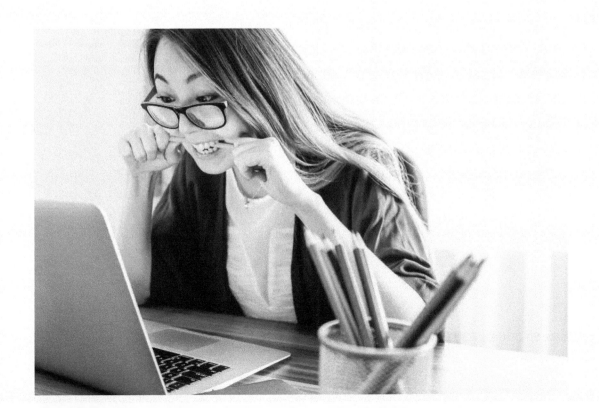

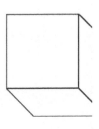

# Incorporating Meditation and Mindfulness into Your Practice

Meditation and mindfulness are essential components of a well-rounded yoga practice. By incorporating these practices into your routine, you can deepen your connection to yourself and the present moment, leading to increased stress relief and spirituality.

Meditation is the practice of quieting the mind and focusing on the breath or a mantra. It allows you to cultivate a sense of inner peace and calm, which can be especially beneficial for those dealing with stress or anxiety. By setting aside just a few minutes each day to meditate, you can improve your mental clarity and emotional well-being. Mindfulness, on the other hand, involves being fully present in the moment and paying attention to your thoughts, feelings, and sensations without judgment. This practice can help you develop a greater sense of self-awareness and compassion towards yourself and others. By incorporating mindfulness into your yoga practice, you can deepen your connection to your body and breath, allowing for a more profound spiritual experience.

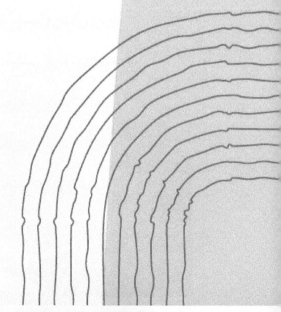

There are many ways to incorporate meditation and mindfulness into your yoga practice. You can start by setting aside a few minutes at the beginning or end of your practice to meditate or practice mindfulness. You can also incorporate mindfulness into your movements by focusing on your breath and body sensations as you move through poses.

Whether you practice hot yoga, aerial yoga, restorative yoga, or any other style, incorporating meditation and mindfulness can enhance your experience and bring a greater sense of peace and spirituality to your practice. So take the time to quiet your mind, be present in the moment, and deepen your connection to yourself through meditation and mindfulness in your yoga practice.

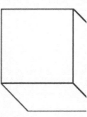

03

# Chapter 3: Yoga for Spirituality

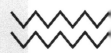

# Connecting Mind, Body, and Spirit through Yoga

In the world of yoga, there is a deep connection between the mind, body, and spirit. Through the practice of yoga, individuals can tap into this powerful connection and achieve a sense of balance and harmony in their lives. In this subchapter, we will explore how yoga can help you connect with your mind, body, and spirit, leading to greater levels of stress relief and spirituality.

Yoga is not just a physical practice; it is a holistic approach to well-being that incorporates elements of mindfulness, meditation, and breathwork. By focusing on the present moment and being fully aware of your body and breath, you can cultivate a sense of inner peace and tranquility. This mindfulness practice can help you to release stress and tension, allowing you to feel more grounded and centered.

Through the physical postures of yoga, you can also connect with your body on a deeper level. By moving your body in new and challenging ways, you can increase flexibility, strength, and balance. This physical awareness can help you to become more in tune with your body's needs and limitations, leading to a greater sense of self-care

Finally, yoga can help you connect with your spirit or inner essence. Through the practice of yoga, you can tap into a sense of spirituality that goes beyond the physical realm. By quieting the mind and tuning into your inner wisdom, you can cultivate a deeper connection with your true self and the world around you.

Whether you are a beginner or an experienced yogi, incorporating yoga into your daily routine can help you to connect with your mind, body, and spirit in a profound way. By embracing the principles of yoga, you can find a sense of peace, balance, and harmony that will benefit every aspect of your life.

# Cultivating a Deeper Sense of Self-Awareness

Cultivating a deeper sense of self-awareness is a key aspect of the transformative practice of yoga. By becoming more attuned to our thoughts, emotions, and physical sensations, we can gain a greater understanding of ourselves and our place in the world. This heightened awareness can lead to increased clarity, inner peace, and a deeper connection to our true selves.

In the fast-paced modern world, it can be easy to lose touch with our inner selves amidst the constant distractions and demands of everyday life. However, by incorporating mindfulness practices into our yoga routine, we can learn to quiet the mind, tune into our bodies, and cultivate a sense of presence and awareness that extends beyond the mat.

One way to deepen our self-awareness through yoga is to focus on the breath. By consciously breathing and paying attention to the breath as it flows in and out of the body, we can anchor ourselves in the present moment and quiet the chatter of the mind. This simple yet powerful practice can help us to become more attuned to our internal state and cultivate a sense of calm and inner peace.

Another way to deepen our self-awareness through yoga is to practice self-reflection and introspection. Taking the time to journal or meditate on our thoughts, emotions, and experiences can help us to gain insight into our patterns, beliefs, and behaviors. By shining a light on our inner world, we can begin to unravel the layers of conditioning and conditioning that may be holding us back from fully embodying our true selves.

Ultimately, cultivating a deeper sense of self-awareness through yoga is a journey of self-discovery and self-realization. By committing to the practice with an open heart and mind, we can tap into our inner wisdom, strength, and resilience, and live more authentically and fully in alignment with our true selves.

# Finding Inner Peace and Harmony through Yoga

Yoga has long been known for its ability to help individuals find inner peace and harmony amidst the chaos of everyday life. Whether you are a seasoned yogi or a beginner, the practice of yoga can provide a sense of calm and tranquility that is essential for maintaining a balanced and centered life.

Through the practice of yoga, individuals can learn to quiet the mind, focus on the present moment, and connect with their inner selves on a deeper level. This connection can help to alleviate stress and anxiety, improve mental clarity, and promote a sense of overall well-being. One of the key ways that yoga helps individuals find inner peace and harmony is through the practice of mindfulness. By focusing on the breath and moving through poses with intention and awareness, individuals can cultivate a sense of presence and mindfulness that can carry over into their daily lives.
In addition to mindfulness, the physical practice of yoga can also help individuals release tension and stress from the body, promoting relaxation and a sense of physical well-being. Whether you prefer the dynamic flow of Vinyasa yoga or the restorative poses of Yin yoga, there is a style of yoga that can help you find the inner peace and harmony you seek.

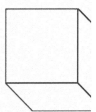

No matter your age or fitness level, yoga can be a powerful tool for finding inner peace and harmony in your life. Whether you are a senior looking to improve flexibility and balance, an athlete seeking to enhance performance and prevent injury, or a beginner just starting your yoga journey, there is a practice that is right for you. Through the practice of yoga, individuals can cultivate a sense of inner peace and harmony that can help them navigate the ups and downs of life with grace and ease. So whether you roll out your mat in a hot yoga studio, hang upside down in an aerial yoga class, or simply find a quiet corner at home to practice, know that the path to inner peace and harmony is always within reach through the practice of yoga.

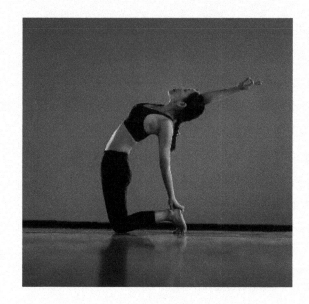

04

# Chapter 4: Specialized Yoga Practices

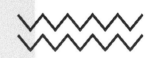

# Hot Yoga: Benefits and Precautions

Hot yoga is a popular form of yoga that involves practicing yoga in a heated room, usually around 95-105 degrees Fahrenheit. This intense practice has gained a following among those looking for a more challenging and detoxifying yoga experience. In this subchapter, we will explore the benefits and precautions of hot yoga for those interested in trying this unique practice.

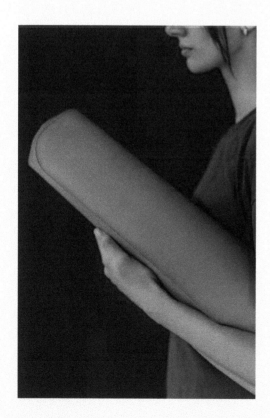

One of the main benefits of hot yoga is its ability to increase flexibility. The heat allows for deeper stretching and helps to loosen tight muscles, making it easier to achieve a greater range of motion. This can be especially beneficial for athletes looking to improve their performance or individuals looking to improve their overall flexibility.

Another benefit of hot yoga is its ability to help with stress relief. The combination of challenging poses and the heat can help to release tension in the body and promote a sense of relaxation. Many practitioners find that hot yoga helps them to clear their minds and focus on the present moment, making it a great practice for those looking to incorporate mindfulness into their daily routine. However, there are some precautions to keep in mind when practicing hot yoga. It is important to stay hydrated before, during, and after class, as the heat can cause you to sweat more than usual. It is also important to listen to your body and take breaks when needed, as the heat can be intense and may lead to overheating if not approached with caution.

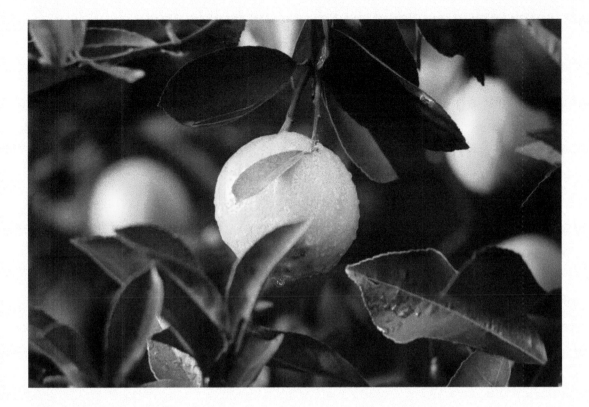

Overall, hot yoga can be a great addition to your yoga practice if you are looking for a challenging and detoxifying experience. Just remember to stay hydrated, listen to your body, and enjoy the benefits of this unique form of yoga.

# Aerial Yoga: Taking Your Practice to New Heights

Aerial yoga is a unique and innovative practice that combines traditional yoga poses with the use of a hammock suspended from the ceiling. This form of yoga allows practitioners to experience the benefits of both yoga and aerial acrobatics, resulting in a fun and challenging workout that can take your practice to new heights – both literally and figuratively.

One of the key benefits of aerial yoga is the decompression of the spine that occurs when practitioners are suspended in the air. This allows for greater flexibility and range of motion, as well as a deeper stretch than traditional yoga poses can provide. In addition, the support of the hammock allows for inversions and other poses that may be difficult or impossible to achieve on the ground, helping to build strength and improve balance.

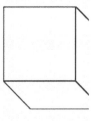

Aerial yoga is also a great way to build core strength, as many poses require engaging the abdominal muscles to stay balanced and supported in the hammock. This can help improve posture and prevent back pain, making it an excellent practice for anyone looking to strengthen their core muscles.

For those interested in deepening their spiritual practice, aerial yoga can also be a powerful tool for cultivating mindfulness and presence. The sensation of floating in the air can help practitioners let go of distractions and focus on the present moment, leading to a greater sense of peace and inner calm.

Whether you are a seasoned yogi looking to shake up your routine or a beginner interested in trying something new, aerial yoga offers a unique and exciting way to take your practice to new heights. So grab a hammock, let go of your fears, and soar into a new realm of physical and spiritual growth with aerial yoga.

# Restorative Yoga: Relaxing and Rejuvenating the Body

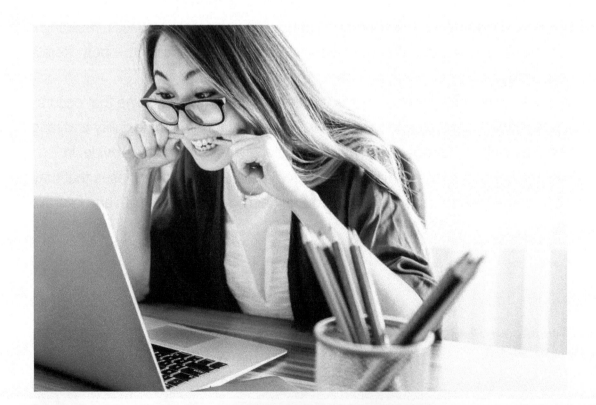

Restorative yoga is a gentle and relaxing form of yoga that focuses on deep relaxation and rejuvenation of the body. It is the perfect practice for those looking to unwind and release stress from their busy lives. Unlike other forms of yoga that may be more physically demanding, restorative yoga is all about slowing down and allowing the body to rest and restore itself.

In restorative yoga, the emphasis is on holding poses for an extended period of time, typically anywhere from 5 to 20 minutes. This allows the body to fully relax and release tension in the muscles. Props such as bolsters, blankets, and blocks are often used to support the body in various poses, making it easier to hold them for longer periods of time.

The benefits of restorative yoga are numerous. Not only does it help to reduce stress and anxiety, but it also promotes deep relaxation and a sense of inner peace. It can also help to improve flexibility, increase circulation, and promote better sleep. For those recovering from injury or illness, restorative yoga can be a gentle way to ease back into a regular yoga practice.

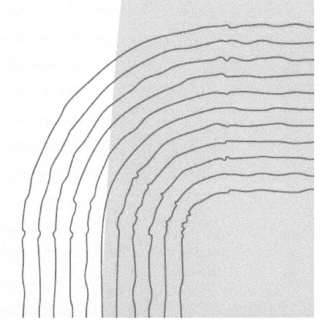

Whether you are new to yoga or a seasoned practitioner, restorative yoga is a wonderful practice to incorporate into your routine. It is especially beneficial for those who may be dealing with chronic pain, fatigue, or emotional imbalances. By taking the time to relax and rejuvenate the body through restorative yoga, you can experience a deeper sense of well-being and connection to your inner self.

05

# Chapter 5: Yoga for Different Audiences

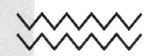

# Yoga for Seniors: Gentle and Safe Practices

As we age, our bodies require more gentle and safe practices to maintain flexibility, balance, and overall well-being. Yoga for seniors focuses on movements and poses that are accessible and beneficial for older adults, taking into consideration any physical limitations or health concerns.

One of the key aspects of yoga for seniors is the emphasis on gentle movements and stretching to improve flexibility and reduce stiffness in the joints. Poses are often modified to accommodate any physical limitations, making them safe and effective for seniors of all levels of fitness.

In addition to physical benefits, yoga for seniors also offers mental and emotional benefits. Through mindfulness and breathwork, seniors can reduce stress, anxiety, and depression, promoting a sense of calm and inner peace.

Incorporating yoga into a senior's routine can also help improve balance and coordination, reducing the risk of falls and injuries. By building strength in the muscles and bones, yoga can help seniors maintain their independence and quality of life as they age.

Some popular yoga practices for seniors include chair yoga, restorative yoga, and gentle yoga. These practices focus on slow, controlled movements and deep breathing to promote relaxation and gentle stretching.

Whether you are a senior looking to improve your physical and mental well-being, or a caregiver looking for ways to support the seniors in your life, yoga for seniors offers a safe and effective way to stay healthy and active in your golden years. Start slowly, listen to your body, and enjoy the many benefits that yoga can bring to your life.

# Yoga for Children: Fun and Playful Poses

Yoga for children is a wonderful way to introduce mindfulness and movement to young ones in a fun and engaging way. In this subchapter, we will explore some playful poses that are perfect for children to practice.

One of the most popular poses for children is the Tree Pose. This pose helps improve balance and focus, while also encouraging a sense of calm and stability. Children can pretend to be trees swaying in the wind, which adds a playful element to the practice.

Another fun pose for children is the Downward Dog. This pose helps stretch the entire body, while also building strength in the arms and legs. Children can pretend to be dogs stretching and wagging their tails, making the pose both enjoyable and beneficial.

The Butterfly Pose is another great option for children. This pose helps open up the hips and improve flexibility in the groin area. Children can flap their "wings" like butterflies while holding this pose, adding a playful touch to their practice.

Lastly, the Warrior Pose is a powerful pose that helps build strength and confidence. Children can pretend to be brave warriors standing strong and tall, embodying the qualities of courage and determination.

Overall, introducing children to yoga at a young age can have numerous benefits for their physical and mental well-being. By incorporating fun and playful poses into their practice, children can develop a love for yoga that will stay with them for years to come. So let's encourage our little ones to get on their mats and explore the wonderful world of yoga!

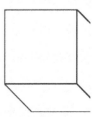

# Prenatal Yoga: Nurturing the Body and Baby

Prenatal yoga is a gentle and safe way for expecting mothers to stay active and healthy during their pregnancy. It focuses on poses and breathing techniques that help to alleviate the aches and pains that can come with carrying a baby, as well as preparing the body for childbirth.

Nurturing the body and baby through prenatal yoga involves connecting with both yourself and your growing baby on a deeper level. The practice encourages mindfulness and relaxation, helping to reduce stress and anxiety that often accompany pregnancy. By focusing on the present moment and your breath, you can create a sense of calm and peace that can benefit both you and your baby.

Prenatal yoga also helps to improve flexibility, strength, and balance, which can be especially beneficial as your body goes through the many changes of pregnancy. It can also help to alleviate common discomforts such as back pain, swollen ankles, and tight hips. By practicing prenatal yoga regularly, you can increase your overall well-being and prepare your body for the physical demands of labor and delivery.

Whether you are new to yoga or have been practicing for years, prenatal yoga offers a unique opportunity to connect with your body, your baby, and your inner self. It is a nurturing and empowering practice that can help you to feel more confident, relaxed, and in tune with your pregnancy journey. So take some time for yourself and your baby, and explore the beauty and benefits of prenatal yoga.

# Yoga for Beginners: Building a Strong Foundation

For those new to the practice of yoga, building a strong foundation is essential for long-term success and growth. Whether you are drawn to yoga for its physical benefits, stress relief, or spiritual connection, establishing a solid base will set you up for a fulfilling and transformative journey.

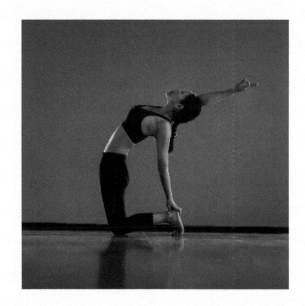

Beginners often feel overwhelmed by the variety of yoga styles and poses available. It is important to remember that everyone's yoga journey is unique, and it is perfectly normal to start slow and gradually progress at your own pace. By focusing on building a strong foundation, you will develop the strength, flexibility, and mindfulness needed to advance in your practice.

One of the key aspects of building a strong foundation in yoga is establishing a consistent practice. Set aside dedicated time each day to practice yoga, even if it is just for a few minutes. Consistency is key to progress, and by making yoga a regular part of your routine, you will begin to see improvements in your physical and mental well-being.

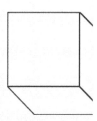

In addition to a consistent practice, beginners should also focus on proper alignment and breathing techniques. Paying attention to alignment will help prevent injuries and ensure that you are getting the most benefit from each pose. Breath awareness is also crucial in yoga, as it helps to calm the mind and deepen your practice.

As you continue to build a strong foundation in your yoga practice, remember to be patient and compassionate with yourself. Progress may be slow at times, but with dedication and perseverance, you will see improvements in your physical, mental, and spiritual well-being. Yoga is a journey of self-discovery and transformation, and by laying a strong foundation, you are setting yourself up for a fulfilling and enriching experience.

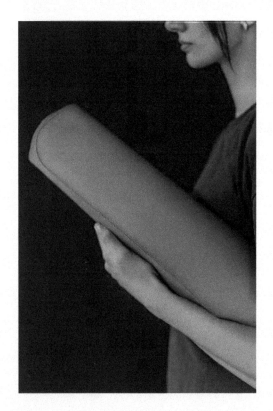

06

# Chapter 6: Advanced Yoga Practices

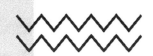

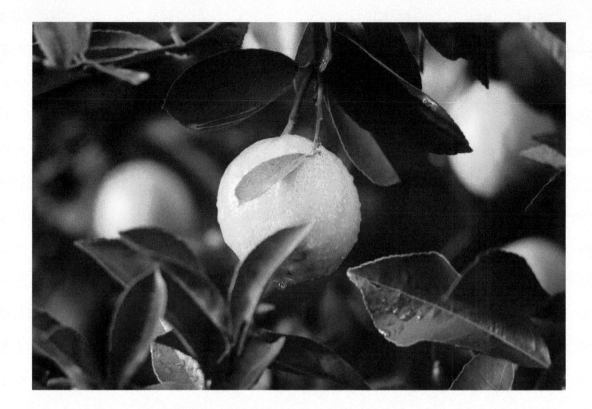

# Vinyasa Yoga: Flowing Sequences for Strength and Flexibility

Vinyasa yoga, also known as "flow" yoga, is a dynamic practice that focuses on linking breath with movement. This style of yoga is perfect for those looking to build strength, increase flexibility, and find a sense of flow and connection in their practice. In this subchapter, we will explore how Vinyasa yoga can help you achieve these goals and more.

Vinyasa yoga sequences are designed to create a seamless flow of movement, allowing you to transition smoothly from one pose to the next. This constant movement and focus on breath help to build heat in the body, promoting strength and endurance. As you move through the poses, you will also work on improving your flexibility, as many Vinyasa sequences incorporate stretches and twists that help to open up tight muscles and joints.

One of the key benefits of Vinyasa yoga is its ability to help you find a sense of mindfulness and presence on the mat. By linking breath with movement, you are encouraged to stay present in the moment, letting go of any distractions or worries outside of the yoga studio. This focus on mindfulness can help to reduce stress and anxiety, promoting a sense of calm and relaxation in both body and mind.

Whether you are new to yoga or a seasoned practitioner, Vinyasa yoga offers something for everyone. Its flowing sequences can be modified to suit any level of experience, making it a versatile practice that can be adapted to meet your individual needs. So, roll out your mat, find your breath, and let the flow of Vinyasa yoga guide you towards strength, flexibility, and a deeper sense of connection with your inner self.

# Yoga for Athletes: Enhancing Performance and Preventing Injuries

In the world of sports and athletics, finding ways to enhance performance and prevent injuries is crucial. Yoga has become increasingly popular among athletes as a way to achieve these goals. The practice of yoga not only improves flexibility, strength, and balance, but also helps athletes develop mental focus and clarity.

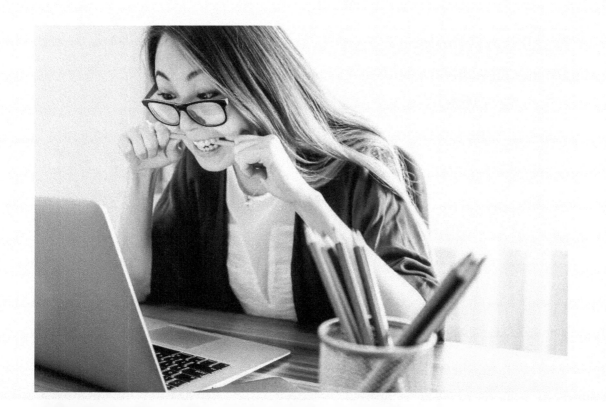

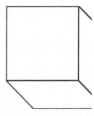

For athletes looking to take their performance to the next level, incorporating yoga into their training regimen can be a game-changer. By practicing yoga regularly, athletes can increase their range of motion, improve their body awareness, and even boost their endurance and stamina. Additionally, yoga can help athletes recover faster from intense workouts and competitions, reducing the risk of overuse injuries.

One of the key benefits of yoga for athletes is its ability to prevent injuries. By strengthening the muscles and joints, improving alignment, and increasing flexibility, yoga can help athletes avoid common injuries like strains, sprains, and tears. The mindfulness aspect of yoga also helps athletes tune into their bodies, allowing them to recognize and address any imbalances or weaknesses before they lead to injury.

Whether you're a professional athlete or a weekend warrior, incorporating yoga into your training routine can have a profound impact on your performance and overall well-being. By practicing yoga for athletes, you can enhance your physical abilities, prevent injuries, and cultivate a deeper sense of mindfulness and focus that can benefit you both on and off the field.

07

# Chapter 7:
# Maintaining a Regular
# Yoga Practice

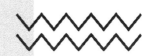

# Setting Realistic Goals and Intentions

Setting realistic goals and intentions is a crucial aspect of any yoga practice, as it helps us stay focused and motivated on our spiritual journey. Whether you are a seasoned yogi or a beginner looking to explore the benefits of yoga, having clear intentions will guide you towards achieving your desired outcomes.

In the world of spirituality, meditation, ZEN, and mindfulness, setting realistic goals can help us stay grounded and connected to our inner selves. By identifying what we hope to achieve through our yoga practice, we can create a roadmap that will lead us towards a more balanced and harmonious life.

For those practicing hot yoga, aerial yoga, restorative yoga, or any other specialized forms of yoga, setting intentions can help us deepen our practice and experience the full benefits of these unique styles. Whether you are looking to build strength, increase flexibility, or simply find inner peace, having clear goals in mind will keep you on track and motivated.

Even for specific niches such as yoga for seniors, yoga for children, vinyasa yoga, yoga for athletes, prenatal yoga, or yoga for stress relief, setting realistic goals is essential. By understanding our limitations and capabilities, we can tailor our practice to suit our individual needs and ensure that we are moving towards our objectives in a safe and sustainable way.

Remember, the key to setting realistic goals and intentions is to be honest with yourself about what you hope to achieve and to be patient with your progress. By staying focused and committed to your practice, you will gradually see the benefits unfold in your mind, body, and soul.

# Overcoming Challenges and Plateaus

In our yoga journey, we often face challenges and plateaus that can hinder our progress and growth. These obstacles can come in many forms, such as physical limitations, mental blocks, or simply a lack of motivation. However, it is important to remember that these challenges are a natural part of the practice and can ultimately lead to greater self-discovery and transformation.

One of the key ways to overcome challenges and plateaus in yoga is to practice mindfulness and self-awareness. By tuning into our bodies and minds during our practice, we can better understand the root causes of our obstacles and work towards finding solutions. This may involve modifying poses to accommodate physical limitations, incorporating breathing techniques to calm the mind, or setting new intentions to reignite our passion for the practice.

Another effective way to overcome challenges in yoga is to seek support from others. Whether it be through attending classes with a supportive community, working with a knowledgeable teacher, or engaging in discussions with fellow practitioners, having a support system can provide us with the encouragement and guidance needed to push through our plateaus.

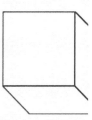

It is also important to remember that progress in yoga is not always linear. There will be times when we feel like we are not making any advancements, but it is during these moments that we must trust in the process and have faith that growth is still occurring, albeit at a slower pace.

By embracing challenges and plateaus in our yoga practice, we can cultivate resilience, patience, and a deeper sense of self-awareness that will ultimately lead to spiritual growth and transformation. Remember, the journey of yoga is not about reaching a destination, but rather about the lessons we learn and the growth we experience along the way.

# Creating a Sacred Space for Your Practice

Creating a sacred space for your yoga practice is essential to deepening your connection with yourself and the divine. Whether you practice yoga for stress relief, spirituality, or mindfulness, having a dedicated space where you can focus and center yourself is crucial.

First and foremost, choose a quiet and clutter-free area in your home where you can practice without distractions. This could be a spare room, a corner of your bedroom, or even a spot in your living room that you can set aside just for your practice. Make sure the space is clean and inviting, with minimal decorations that are calming and inspiring.

Next, consider adding elements that enhance the sacredness of your space. This could include burning incense or sage, playing soft music, or lighting candles to create a peaceful ambiance. You may also want to incorporate items that hold personal significance to you, such as crystals, mala beads, or photos of loved ones.

When practicing in your sacred space, make sure to set intentions for your practice and take a few moments to center yourself before beginning. This could involve deep breathing, meditation, or simply closing your eyes and tuning in to your body and breath.

By creating a sacred space for your practice, you are setting the stage for a deeper and more meaningful experience on the mat. Whether you are practicing hot yoga, restorative yoga, vinyasa yoga, or any other style, having a dedicated space where you can connect with yourself and the divine will enhance your practice and bring greater peace and clarity to your life.

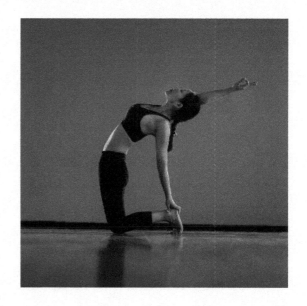

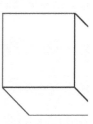

08

# Chapter 8: The Spiritual Journey of Yoga

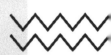

# Embracing the Present Moment with Mindfulness

In today's fast-paced world, it can be easy to get caught up in the hustle and bustle of daily life, constantly worrying about the future or dwelling on the past. However, embracing the present moment with mindfulness is a powerful practice that can help alleviate stress and bring a sense of peace and clarity to your life.

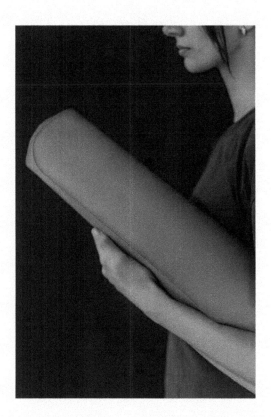

Mindfulness is the practice of being fully present in the moment, without judgment or attachment to the past or future. By focusing on the here and now, you can cultivate a sense of awareness and appreciation for the present moment, allowing you to fully experience life as it unfolds.

Yoga is a powerful tool for cultivating mindfulness, as it encourages you to focus on your breath, body, and sensations during each pose. By practicing yoga with mindfulness, you can learn to tune into your body's signals, release tension and stress, and connect with your inner self on a deeper level. Whether you prefer hot yoga, aerial yoga, restorative yoga, or vinyasa yoga, incorporating mindfulness into your practice can enhance the benefits of each session. By approaching each pose with awareness and intention, you can deepen your mind-body connection and experience a greater sense of peace and tranquility.

Mindfulness is not just beneficial on the yoga mat - it can also be applied to all aspects of your life. By bringing mindfulness into your daily routine, you can cultivate a sense of gratitude, compassion, and acceptance for yourself and others.

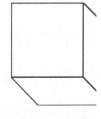

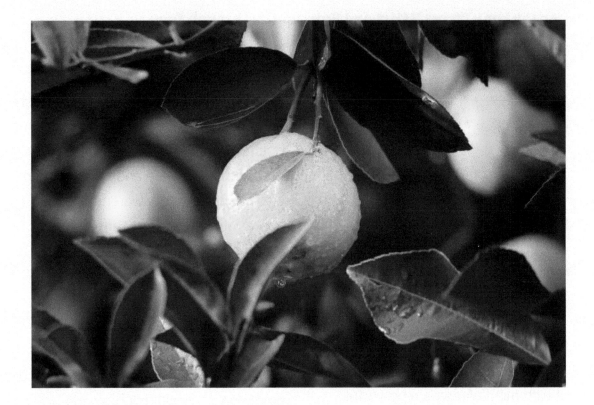

So take a moment to pause, breathe, and embrace the present moment with mindfulness. By incorporating this practice into your yoga routine and daily life, you can find greater peace, clarity, and joy in each moment.

# Cultivating a Sense of Gratitude and Compassion

In the fast-paced world we live in, it can be easy to get caught up in the chaos and forget to take a moment to appreciate the little things in life. Cultivating a sense of gratitude and compassion through yoga can help us slow down, connect with our inner selves, and find peace amidst the storm.

Practicing yoga is not just about physical exercise; it is also a spiritual practice that can help us tap into our emotions and cultivate a sense of gratitude for all that we have. By focusing on our breath, moving mindfully through poses, and taking the time to appreciate our bodies and minds, we can begin to shift our perspective and see the beauty in every moment.

Gratitude is a powerful tool that can help us find joy and contentment in our lives, no matter what challenges we may be facing. When we take the time to acknowledge all the blessings we have, big and small, we can cultivate a sense of peace and fulfillment that will carry us through even the toughest of times.

Compassion is another important aspect of yoga that can help us connect with others and foster a sense of community and understanding. By practicing loving-kindness meditation and sending positive energy to those around us, we can open our hearts and minds to the beauty and diversity of the world.

Whether you are a seasoned yogi or a beginner just starting out on your journey, incorporating gratitude and compassion into your practice can help you deepen your spiritual connection and find true inner peace. Take the time to reflect on all that you have to be grateful for, and let that gratitude guide you as you move through your practice and your life.

# Finding Peace and Harmony Within Yourself and the World

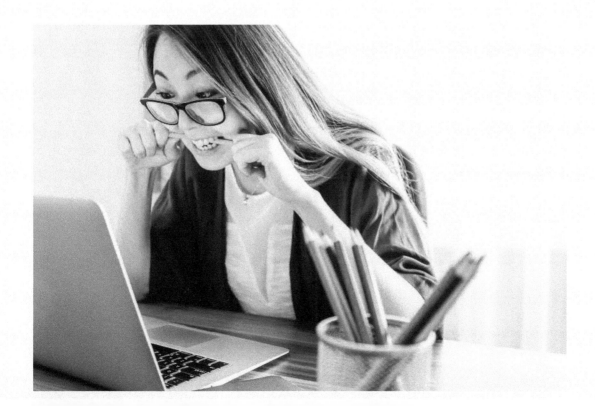

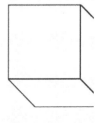

In the fast-paced and chaotic world we live in, finding peace and harmony within ourselves and the world around us can seem like an impossible task. However, through the practice of yoga, we can cultivate a sense of calm and tranquility that can help us navigate through life's challenges with grace and ease.

Yoga is not just a physical practice; it is also a spiritual one that can help us connect with our inner selves and the world around us. By focusing on our breath and being present in the moment, we can let go of stress and anxiety and find a sense of peace within ourselves.

Practicing yoga can also help us cultivate a sense of harmony with the world around us. By honoring our bodies and treating ourselves with kindness and compassion, we can extend that same love and care to others and the planet. Through mindfulness and awareness, we can become more attuned to the needs of those around us and work towards creating a more peaceful and harmonious world.

Whether you are a beginner or an experienced yogi, there are many different styles of yoga that can help you find peace and harmony within yourself and the world. From restorative yoga for relaxation to vinyasa yoga for strength and flexibility, there is a practice that can meet you where you are and help you on your journey towards inner peace and harmony.

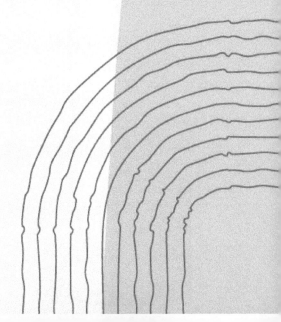

By incorporating yoga into your daily routine, you can tap into a sense of spirituality and mindfulness that can help you navigate through life's ups and downs with grace and ease. So take a deep breath, roll out your mat, and let the practice of yoga guide you towards finding peace and harmony within yourself and the world.

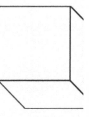

Milton Keynes UK
Ingram Content Group UK Ltd.
UKHW052037100324
439157UK00007B/22